ATTAINING HEALTH
Through
Salah & Ablution

ATTAINING HEALTH
Through
Salah & Ablution

Anayat Bukhari

To order additional copies of this book, contact:
Xlibris
1-800-455-039
www.Xlibris.com.au
Orders@Xlibris.com.au
717950

LIST OF CONTENTS

BOOK REVIEW

It is my privilege to be able to write a review on 'Attaining Health through Salah and Ablution' by Anayat Bukhari.

The Author has indeed chosen to include the physical benefits, which are seldom emphasised whilst discussing the spiritual benefits of Salah (compulsory ritualistic prayer in Islam).

Being a Psychiatrist, I am particularly impressed by the psychological and mental effects mentioned by the Author especially highlighting the benefits starting from intention of prayer and continuing effects afterwards.

The most fascinating thing about this book is how the author has shared his own personal experiences and long lasting effects of Salah. In the end, effects of Salah in one's life in general are highlighted making this book a complete reference for such topic.

I would highly recommend this book for not only those who have interest in health, fitness and spirituality but also those who may be intrigued about religion affecting a person's life in various domains.

Dr Fawaz Mufti,
Psychiatrist,
Gold Coast, Australia

AUTHOR BIOGRAPHY

Anayat Bukhari is an award-winning author (I.I.University Islamabad 1994). He has a passion for writing on diverse subjects. At a very young age, he started transferring his thoughts on the paper in the form of short essays and prose.

With growing age, his selection of topics became more mature, and he started to focus on serious social, moral, political, lifestyle, and spiritual subjects.

He is not your normal fiction writer. His unique selection of topics, in-depth research, and comprehensive but simple explanation of complex realities makes his work interesting to read. His philosophy regarding life and spirituality, when transferred into words, creates literature that stands out among today's modern literature.

https://au.linkedin.com/pub/anayat-bukhari/2a/914/b04

FOREWORD

I usually come across the people suffering from musculoskeletal problems at different occasions. Most of them receive advice from their Medical men to perform certain exercises to address their issue. Many countries have developed a full network for body fitness in the form of a huge business. People spend huge amounts and spare time to keep fit but still they suffer a lot. This led me to conceive the idea to explore a simple, easy and practicable way to keep fit.

The quest of easy path to fitness made me search through various options. Traditional exercises, Yoga, Diet supplements, Sports, etc. all are different methods to keep your body fit. Each of them has some complication or limitation which renders it unpractical for the common man. I found a lot of stuff on the Medical and physical benefits of Wudu and Salah in a scattered form. I decided to compile it in a comprehensive form to create a formal guideline for the benefit of general public. Studying this booklet can be beneficial both for Muslims and non-Muslims. It is tried to present authentic information only to substantiate the benefits of various movements in salah and different segments of ablution. Anyhow, any error pointed out will be appreciated.

References are provided in the text and terminology is elaborated in the footings. Suggestions will also be welcomed to improve the work at a level to make it more beneficial.

Regards
Anayat Bukhari
E. mail: anayatbukhari@yahoo.com

INTRODUCTION

Purity in Islam is of significant importance and there are many verses about purity in Quran. In chapter Maida there is an explicit and direct injunction about purification in Verse 6.

O ye who believe! When ye prepare for Prayer, wash your faces and your hands (and arms) to the elbows; rub your heads (with water) and wash your feet to the Ankles[1]. If ye are in a state of ceremonial impurity [2] Bathe your whole body. But if ye are ill or on a journey or one of you cometh from the privy or ye have been in contact with women and ye find no water then take for yourselves Clean sand or earth, and rub therewith your faces and hands[3]. Allah doth not wish to place you in a difficulty, but (wish) to make you clean and to complete His favor to you that ye may be grateful.

Al-Maida 5, V 6

---

[1] Washing feet without ankles make wudu null and void. According to a Hadis in Muslim Jabir (R.A) reported: Umar b. Khattab said that a person performed ablution and left a small part equal to the space of a nail (unwashed). The Apostle of Allah (Peace be upon Him) saw that and said: Go back and perform ablution well. He then went back (performed ablution well) and offered the prayer.

[2] This is the impurity which arises from sex pollution.

[3] It is termed Tayamum in Islamic Jurisprudence.

So the state of purity is mandatory for Salah (prayer) along with certain other acts of worship. There are several Ahadis pertaining to purification and its importance. Here a few are being mentioned.

> **Abu Malik al-Ashari reported: The Messenger of Allah (Peace be upon Him) said: Cleanliness is half faith and al-Hamdu Lillah (praise be to Allah) fills the scale, and Subhan Allah (glory be to Allah) and al-Hamdu Lillah (praise be to Allah) fill what is in between the heavens and earth, and prayer is a light, and charity is proof (of one's faith) and endurance is a brightness and the Holy Quran is a proof on or against you. All men go out early in the morning and sell themselves, thereby setting themselves free or destroying themselves.**
>
> **Sahih Muslim[4]**

There is another Hadis which tells us that ablution is essential for prayer.

> **Hammam bin Munabbih, who is the brother of Wahb bin Munabbih, said: This is what has been transmitted to us by Abu Huraira from Muhammad, the Messenger of Allah (Peace be upon Him), and then narrated ahadis out of them and observed that the Messenger of Allah (Peace be upon Him) said: The prayer of none amongst you would be accepted in a state of impurity till he performs ablution.[5]**
>
> **Sahih Muslim[6]**

To attain purity, a Muslim has to take bath if the Ritual impurity arises from sex pollution[7]. For prayers ritual ablution (wudu) is essential. It includes washing of face, both hands along with arms

---

[4] Sahih Muslim- Kitab Al-Taharah Chapter XCIII - 432
[5] This Hadis makes it clear that wudu (ablution) is obligatory for prayer.
[6] Sahih Muslim - Kitab Al-Taharah, Chapter XCIV - 435
[7] Sex pollution has a lot of detail which can be seen in books of Ahadis and Islamic Jurisprudence.

with elbows, wiping of head with wet hands and the washing of feet including ankles. In addition to these, rinsing the mouth cavity and cleaning the inner side of the nose and wiping of ears & neck is also practiced as to follow the Sunnah[8] of Prophet Muhammad (Peace be upon Him).

There is a choice to attain purity by using dirt with certain conditions. First, when water is not available and the second when the water is there but it is harmful to use due to illness.

Salah (prayer) five times a day is the second pillar[9] of Islam. It has been mentioned about seven hundred times in Quran. Out of these, sixty times there are clear injunctions about Salah. We will present here a few verses to explain the point.

> **And be steadfast in prayer; give Zakat and bow down your heads with those, who bow down (in worship).**
>
> **Al-Baqarah 2, V 43**

> **Guard strictly, your (habit of) prayers. Especially the Middle Prayer and stand[10] before Allah in a devout (frame of mind).**
> **Al-Baqarah 2, V 238**

> **Successful indeed are the Believers, who humble themselves[11] in their Prayer.**
> **Al-Muminun 23, V 1-2**

---

[8] Acts that the Holy Prophet (Peace be upon Him) did.

[9] There are five pillars of Islam; Creed of faith-Tauheed(oneness), salah, zakat, fasting and Hajj.

[10] The Middle prayer has been translated from Salatul wusta. There are several interpretations regarding it but most of the scholars are of the view that it is about Asr (in afternoon). This is apt to be most neglected and yet this is the most necessary, to remind us of Allah in the midst of our worldly affairs.

[11] Humility in prayer as regards; estimate of their own worth in Allah's presence, estimate of their own powers & strength and the petitions they offer to Allah.

Recite what is sent of the Book by inspiration to thee, and establish Regular Prayer; for Prayer restrains from shameful and evil deeds[12]. And remembrance of Allah is the greatest (thing in life) without doubt. And Allah knows the (deeds) that ye do.

Al-Ankabut 29, V 45

These verses are enough to clarify the significance of Salah. There are certain mental, oral and physical actions which jointly make this spiritual worship possible. Obviously all the acts of worship have certain rewards from Almighty Allah and Salah is not an exception. Every Muslim has the belief that any good deed in response to the commandment of Allah has certain virtue and any prohibition that is followed by a Muslim is a virtue along with wisdom.

Spiritual benefits[13] of Salah are vastly discussed subject and most of the Muslims are aware of it. Unfortunately, the physical benefits[14] attached to Salah and Ablution is not given the required importance. Hence, majority of the Muslims don't know much about the Medical aspect of these great acts of worship.

Being a Muslim we do believe that wudu has many spiritual benefits apart from its physical benefits. So how can it be possible that a great icon of worship – salah carry only spiritual benefits and is devoid of any physical benefits?

The objective of this book is to highlight the physical benefits of Salah and Ablution by a special focus on Medical aspect of these acts of worship. Thanks to Almighty Allah; I have been practicing wudu, and salah for about fifty years and have experienced their effects on my body. I also saw the people who do not practice it at

---

[12] Establishing regular prayer is helpful in restraining from sins and evil deeds. Scholars commented on it that if your salah is not doing so then improve the quality of your salah, until you achieve this standard.

[13] The aim and objective of salah is spiritual benefits because we establish salah to obey the commandments of Allah. This obedience is just to please Allah and makes us worthy to get rewards of Allah.

[14] Although physical benefits of prayer and ablution are not the objective of a true Muslim but having its knowledge, certainly is an encouragement for a believer as well as for non-believer. It comes as a bonus with the actual spiritual benefits of salah and a bounty of Allah Almighty.

all through out their lives. I also got an opportunity to observe closely the lives of the people who practice these randomly. Visiting different Masajid for congregational salah provided me the opportunity to closely observe the salah related activities of hundreds of people and its effects on their physical fitness. Here in this booklet I'll try to share my experience so that others can also achieve benefits by practicing wudu and salah regularly. Certain conclusions of various studies are also mentioned in this booklet to add more for the benefit of my readers. It is tried to present the facts with authentic studies only. Some details are the outcome of commonsense and every one can verify these by using wisdom. Having the knowledge of physical benefits will be helpful to get encouraged to perform Salah and Ablution with more devotion and sincerity, in sha Allah.

May Allah bestow upon me the wisdom to make this book most useful and inspiring for the readers to follow the right path, Aameen.

ABLUTION

This is an act of attaining physical purity of certain body parts, which are most exposed to the environment, by using water. These parts are hands, face, head and feet. There is a natural consensus over the fact that washing with water cleans and cleaning means less germs. Lesser germs mean less chances of being prone to various diseases. Less chance of disease means good health. This is the simple physical philosophy of ablution. Now we will take each step of ablution separately to check it in detail.

a- Hands:

- Washing hands before starting Ablution (wudu) makes sure that the hands will be clean when touching other body parts while performing wudu. It lessens the danger of transmitting any germs to other parts through hands. Hands are the most prone part of the body to germs as they touch every thing in daily life. Common infections through dirty hands are; acute respiratory infections, helminthes (parasitic worm) infection, eye infection & diarrheal disease[15].
- Secondly, hands are comprised of too many bones and joints to make it flexible. When we wash our hands we constantly move them in different angles, which is a very useful exercise of the joints and their muscles. This exercise helps them to stay healthy as one of the most used part of the body.

---

[15] The Medical benefits of ablution; Ummah 1 TV, Posted 14.09.2011 (contents extracted)

- In 2007 an article was published in British Medical Journal which says, that physical barriers to infection (i.e. hand washing) if given more of a priority can be more effective than drugs[16].
- A study carried out in Pakistan found that over 50% of Pneumonia related infections in children under the age of 5 could simply be prevented by developing the habit of washing hands with soup. Hand wash reduces respiratory infections by removing infectious pathogens to be found on the hands[17].
- There are three major veins passing through arms to the Heart, Liver and Brain. Rubbing the arms while washing them stimulates these veins which results in increase the flow of blood towards these organs[18].

b- Face:

- Face is the host of all the five sensory organs – ears, eyes, nose, tongue and skin. These organs can catch infection through unclean and full of germs face. Their performance is much enhanced by washing the face through a regular system of ablution.
- Apart from cleaning, the face washing is also responsible to recharge different organs such as intestines, stomach and bladder[19].
- Regular washing of face at intervals put positive effect on Nervous system and Reproductive system.
- The beauty and freshness of face increases by regular washing at intervals with water[20].

---

16   The Medical benefits of ablution; Ummah 1 TV, Posted 14.09.2011 (contents extracted)

17   The Medical benefits of ablution; Ummah 1 TV, Posted 14.09.2011 (contents extracted)

18   The Medical benefits of ablution; Ummah 1 TV, Posted 14.09.2011 (contents extracted)

19   Dr. Magomedov, assistant to the department of the man's general hygiene and ecology in Daghestan State Medical Academy.

20   Prayers: a sport for the body and soul. By Mukhtar Salem

c- Head:

- The head is connected to the body through neck. All the veins and the arteries pass through neck and the skull is also littered with these veins and arteries which run throughout the body, to the brain and to the spinal cord. The wiping of the head and the back area of the neck including ears with wet hands stimulate these veins and arteries. It results in increase in blood flow and strengthens these organs[21].
- Generous wiping of the head by wet hands keeps the scalp fresh by reducing dandruff which makes hair stay longer than average.
- Wiping of ears with wet fingers keep the ears from dirt on the outer ear to enter it and become wax which leads to ear infection and results in imbalance of the body.

d- Feet:

- Feet are considered the most neglected part of the body and it is observed that a large number of healthy people also have various issues with their feet. Most common among these are fungal problems (athlete's foot) and crack heals apart from other hygiene related infections. Regular washing of feet daily during ablution keeps them fit.
- The National Diabetes Information Clearinghouse (NDIC) recommends to the patients of Diabetes to keep the skin of feet healthy. One way being washing your feet in warm water every day[22].
- Feet are washed including certain part of legs – ankles[23]. An expert of Chinese way of treatment Dr. Magomedov confirms

---

[21] The Medical benefits of ablution; Ummah 1 TV, Posted 14.09.2011
[22] The Medical benefits of ablution; Ummah 1 TV, Posted 14.09.2011
[23] A Hadis in Sahih Muslim, Kitab Al-Taharah – Nauman b. Abdullah reported: He saw Abu Huraira (R.A) perform ablution. He washed his face and washed his hands up to the arms. He then washed his feet and reached up to the shanks, and then said: I heard Allah's Messenger (Peace be upon Him) say: My people would come with bright faces and bright hands and feet on account of the marks of

that by washing right leg during wudu we reach, to strengthen the osseous system (skeleton), intestine, nervous system, lumbar area, stomach, pancreas, gall bladder, thyroid gland and others, through the Biologically Active Spots (BAS).

- Washing left foot we stimulate BAS responsible for the working of pituitary gland located in the brain. It regulates the function of endocrine glands to control the growth[24].

e- Mouth:

- Rinsing of mouth cavity is Sunnah during wudu. Certainly it helps to clean the mouth by removing unwanted food particles, some germs and oral odour. Washing mouth cavity along with Miswak and gargling is an excellent way to maintain oral hygiene.
- Holy Prophet (Peace be upon Him) emphasized on using Miswak (Tooth stick) during wudu. There are several Ahadis pertaining to tooth stick, one of these is as follows:

> **Abu Huraira reported: The Apostle (Peace be upon Him) said: Were it not that I might overburden the believers—and in the Hadis transmitted by Zuhair "people"---I would have ordered them to use tooth stick at every time of prayer.**
>
> **Sahih Muslim[25]**

- Miswak is recommended several times i.e. before leaving on a journey, before entering the home after returning from a journey, before sleeping, after waking up and before prayer.
- Miswak is an effective tool for cleaning mouth due to its antiseptic properties. It helps to halt tooth decay, reduces plaque and gingivitis by abolishing harmful germs of the mouth. The World Health Organization (WHO) in year

---

ablution, so he who can increase the luster of his forehead (and that of his hands and legs) should do so.

[24] Dr. Magomed Magomedov, assistant to the Department of man's general hygiene and ecology in Daghestan State Medical Academy.

[25] Kitab Al-Taharah, Chapter CII - 487

2000 backed an internal consensus on using the Miswak to Improve oral hygiene[26].

- Although tooth brush is being used vastly in the modern world but a scientific study in 2003 concluded, "The Miswak is more effective then tooth brushing for reducing plaque and gingivitis when preceded by professional instruction in its correct application"[27].
- A clean mouth is certainly helpful in maintaining body hygiene as most of the germs pass on to the stomach through unclean mouth.

f- Nose[28]:

- Washing the inner part of the nose and blowing it out removes dirt and mucous from the nostrils which maintains respiratory tract regularly. Obviously a clean Trachea helps sufficient supply of Oxygen to the body through lungs. This is another phenomenon which contributes to the health of the body.
- It is a good and easy prevention from dust and pollen allergy, which lead to flu, soar throat and sometimes fever[29].

---

[26] The Medical benefits of ablution; Ummah 1 TV, Posted 14.09.2011 (contents extracted)

[27] The Medical benefits of ablution; Ummah 1 TV, Posted 14.09.2011 (contents extracted)

[28] Hammam b. Munabbih reported: This is what Abu Huraira transmitted to us from Muhammad, The Messenger of Allah (Peace be upon Him) and he mentioned a number of Ahadis, of which this is one that The Messenger of Allah (Peace be upon Him) said: When anyone amongst you (performs ablution) he must snuff his nostrils with water and then clean them.........Sahih Muslim – Kitab Al Taharah, Chapter XCVII - 459

[29] Study conducted by a team of Doctors of Alexandria University, The Prophetic Tradition, which urges the exaggeration of washing the nostrils by introducing the water in the nostrils and then blowing it out, in the correct form had clean, shiny nostrils with no dust clinging to the small hair inside the nostril. Those who did not perform ablution had light colored, greasy nostrils and their hair of nostrils fell off easily.

How to perform Ablution?

Quran mentions only four body parts to be washed. But the detail of performing wudu, can be find only in Ahadis, just like the elaboration of salah, zakah, etc. There is a long hadis in Muslim which relates the complete method of performing wudu:

> **Humran, the freed slave of Uthman, said: Uthman b. Affan called for ablution water and this is how he performed the ablution. He washed his hands thrice. He then rinsed his mouth and cleaned his nose with water (three times). He then washed his face three times, then washed his right arm[30] up to the elbow three times, then washed his left arm like that, then wiped his head; then washed his right foot up to the ankle three times, then washed his left foot like that, and the said: I saw the Messenger of Allah (Peace be upon Him) said: He who performs ablution like this ablution of mine and then stood up (for prayer) and offered two Rakah (unit) of prayer without allowing his thoughts to be distracted, all his previous sins are expiated. Ibn Shihab said: Our scholars remarked: This is the most complete of the ablutions performed for prayer.**
>
> **Sahih Muslim[31]**

Ablution and Chinese Treatment

Dr. Magomedov- an expert of Chinese treatment[32] says that there are more than 700 Biologically Active Spots (BAS) in a human body. Sixty six of them have quick reflex therapy effects and are

---

[30] Starting from the right hand side for ablution. Ayesha (R.A) reported: The Messenger of Allah (Peace be upon Him) loved to start from the right-hand side for performing ablution, for combing (the hair) and wearing the shoes. Sahih Muslim; Kitab Al-Taharah, Chapter CV - 514

[31] Kitab Al-Taharah, Chapter XCV - 436

[32] Dr. Magomed Magomedov, Assistant to the department of the man's General Hygiene and ecology in the Daghestan State Medical Academy

named the drastic spots or prime elements. Sixty one of these are located in the zones which are required to wash in wudu while the other five are located between the ankle and knee.

Dr. Magomedov said that his studies were triggered by his solemn belief that the five time a day prayers were bound to have not only an indisputable spiritual effect but were also bound to have a purely physical healing effect[33].

Staying in Wudu

Normally every Muslim performs wudu at least twice a day to offer his prayers but it may increase up to five times. This is not the limit as staying in wudu is itself an act of worship and it is rewarded by Allah Almighty[34]. For this purpose we perform a new wudu whenever it comes to an end. Allah has praised people who stay pure several times in Quran.

To perform wudu before going to sleep is encouraged by the Holy Prophet (pbuh). According to Him (pbuh) a person who died in the state of wudu will be among the Martyrs on resurrection. Although sleep is a breaker of wudu but going to sleep in the state of wudu is enough to grab this reward[35].

This emphasis on staying in wudu is supported by the Yoga experts. According to them washing important motor and sensory organs such as hands, arms, eyes, legs, mouth and genitals before sleep, using cold water relaxes the body and prepares it for a deep sleep[36].

---

[33] Dr. Magomed Magomedov, assistant to the Department of the man's general hygiene and ecology in Daghestan State Medical Academy.

[34] The commandment of wudu before establishing salah (Maida 5, V6) in Quran is an explicit injunction. It means that it is obligatory and salah is not accepted without wudu. Allah rewards His slaves for fulfilling every commandment. So the state of wudu is itself a virtue, no matter how long it may be.

[35] Sunni Forum: The preventive and healing wonders of wudu.

[36] Sunniforum: The preventive and healing wonders of wudu. (contents extracted)

Performing wudu several times a day keeps different body parts engaged in movements at different angles for a certain time with suitable intervals. This movement of the body parts, joints and muscles is a constant light exercise of the body. Light exercise with suitable intervals is good to keep fit without overburdening the body.

Wudu also provides relief in high blood pressure by lowering the body temperature to a certain extent. It is the reason that Holy Prophet (Peace be upon Him) has suggested the person in anger to perform wudu.

Physical philosophy of compulsory bath

Many people raise the question about the mandatory (compulsory) bath. They can't satisfy their minds without an apparent link between seminal discharge and bathing. For a Muslim having strong belief, being an injunction of Islam is sufficient to follow it[37]. But for others Scientists have discovered something amazing about compulsory bath[38].

Studies of Scientists say that there are two nervous networks within the human body which regulates all the body functions. One

---

[37] Anas b. Malik reported: A woman asked the Messenger of Allah (Peace be upon Him) about a woman who sees in her dream what a man sees in his dream (sexual dream). He (the Holy Prophet) said: If she experiences what a man experiences, she should take a bath........... Sahih Muslim – Kitab Al-Taharah, chapter CXXIV – 609

Aisha (R.A) reported: When Allah's Messenger (Peace be upon Him) bathed because of sexual intercourse, he first washed his hands: he then poured water with his right hand on his left hand and washed his private parts. He then performed ablution as is done for prayer. He then took some water and put his fingers and moved them through the roots of his hair. And when he found that these had been properly moistened, then poured three handfuls on his head and then poured water over his body and subsequently washed his feet........Sahih Muslim – Kitab Al-Taharah, chapter CXXVI - 616

[38] Ghusl after Intercourse: Why? / www.Islamonline.net
    www.med-health.net
    Sex and the Nervous System by Walnut Creak Chiropractor Blog | Dr. David Ritchie DC

of these is Sympathetic nerves and the second is Para-sympathetic nerves. The first one accelerates the activities of various tracts of the body and the second performs the role of brakes. It keeps balance in the function of the body[39].

At times of certain occurrences in the body this balance is disrupted – one of these is "orgasm" which is usually contemporaneous with a seminal discharge. The use of water on the body during bath re-establishes the lost equilibrium by the act of orgasm, which is felt in all parts of the body.

In addition to it the compulsory bath also maintains the cleanliness of the body and observance of hygiene throughout the life[40].

This phenomenon is normally the result of close contact of two bodies. It can transfer germs and parasites mutually. Ghusal (Compulsory bath) removes this effect from both of them.

Wudu; a virtual Lock

I feel my body fortified in the state of wudu which keeps me not only from committing sins but also from attack of many kind of germs. By the Grace of Allah; I never experienced a serious sickness in my life. Most of the regular congregational prayer fellows of mine are also enjoying a healthy life. Despite many disparities in eating habits, meal contents and weather changes most of the people remained healthy. The only thing common was regular performing of wudu which played its due role by keeping us all healthy for a long period[41].

---

[39]   Walnut Creek Chiropractor Blog |Dr. David Ritchie DC

[40]   The secret of, Take a Bath for Health; prasetio30.hubpages.com

[41]   We often see a few Mussalis sitting on chairs beside the walls almost in every Masjid. Someone may take it mistakenly as a sick due to salah. It is not so. No one ever experienced joint problems exclusively due to establishing salah, according to my limited knowledge. These people have diverse backgrounds of their present sickness.

  I experienced knee swelling due to exertion in walking on steep surfaces. It was recovered in a couple of weeks as I stopped to walk on steep ways and continued to establish my routine prayers. Alhamd o lillah. (Author's comment)

Performing wudu is a diverting point for the traffic passing through mind as it suspends the worldly thoughts for a certain period and focus it on the act of obedience and submission to Allah. Thus enables the mind to get relieved from stress and anxiety which is extremely helpful in enhancing the efficiency of brain.

Objection can be raised on the factor which played its role to keep all of us healthy but in the absence of any other common factor the validity of this objection becomes null and void. Sickness due to an accident or due to food poisoning can not be included in this category because their origin is different.

SALAH

Salah is an Arabic word. In English it is called prayer and other languages also have specific words for it, but salah being an Arabic word is universally recognized by Muslim community. According to Oxford English Dictionary, it means to address a prayer to God or other deity. Salah also has the meaning of goodness, righteousness and godliness. In Islamic terminology Salah has very broad meaning. When Muslims establish salah, it is not merely an act of worship because during this act they ask from Allah, thanks Him, praise Him and receive guidance from Him. It is a sort of training for the believers to seek multi-dimensional benefits. Human mind can't reach to all the attributes attached to this bounty of Almighty Allah. The emphasis on establishing prayer in Quran[42] is enough to understand that there is some great wisdom[43] behind this pillar of Islam. The Holy Prophet (Peace be upon Him) has intensified it by His words:

---

[42] Salah is the second pillar of Islam, after Oneness of Allah. Salah is mentioned in Quran about seven hundred times in short or detailed forms but there are about sixty places where clear commandments are given to establish salah.

[43] This wisdom can not be confined only to the spiritual attributes of salah as we believe that Islam is a complete way of life to be followed for a successful living in the world and hereafter. Therefore, it must be inclusive to spiritual and physical benefits for a Mussali.

It is narrated on the authority of Jabir (R.A) that he heard the Apostle (Peace be upon Him) saying: Verily between man and between polytheism and unbelief is the negligence of prayer.

Sahih Muslim – Kitab Al-Iman, chapter XXXVI - 146

It is in fact a special type of programming which conditions their body with the help of different physical postures[44]. This conditioning process has a range of effects on the body of the Mussali. That's why **Ibn e Maja** reports a Hadis of Holy Prophet PBUH that salah is a cure for many diseases. Quran has also pointed towards such effects.

Recite what is sent of the book by inspiration to Thee, and establish regular prayer: for regular prayer restrains from shameful and evil deeds.
Al- ankabut 29, V 45

There is another verse in Holy Quran:

And be steadfast in prayer and give zakat: And whatever good ye send forth for your souls before you, ye shall find it with Allah: for Allah sees well all that ye do[45].
Al-Baqarah 2, V110

"Ye shall find it with Allah" are the words which might include physical, psychological and spiritual effects[46]. In these pages, focus is only on the physical and psychological benefits.

---

[44] Offering prayers need certain postures during proceedings; standing, bowing, bending down and sitting, etc.

[45] The universality of the words in this verse are witness to the fact that Mussali will find spiritual, physical or any other benefits just like in paying zakat. Payer of zakat will not get reward only but will also have barakah /flourish in his wealth.

[46] Although a Muslim establishes salah in conformity with the orders of Allah, hoping to please Him and get a reward for it, but physical or any

Alhamd o lillah, I started offering prayers in such an early age that I don't remember when it was[47]. I'm so grateful to Almighty Allah who granted me the ability to offer my prayers regularly up till now and I beseech His permission to do so throughout my life. It was purely due to the Taufiq (capability) given by Allah and the religious environment of my home. I used to change my dwelling several times in my life period and thus I changed several Masaajid to offer congregational salah. Thus I got the opportunity to have maximum prayer fellows with friendly terms with most of them. In this regard I also observed the effects of regular salah on their bodies. It was also natural to compare their physical condition with those who were not as regular as they. Although there is no data of these Mussalies[48] with regular entries but a general estimation by regular observation becomes more authentic if there is consistence.

Now I'll try to elaborate different effects of salah on Mussali. I'll put these in different categories to make it easy to describe and understand.

Psychological &Mental effects[49]

Right from the start of ablution, a state of mind is developed in the performer which is inclusive of concentration on the act of obedience and submission to one supreme power – Allah. Now the mind is put to rest from the worldly affairs which relieves it from stress, anxiety and distraction. Thus impact of this relaxed brain on

---

other benefits are there as the part of package and a bonus. So we should thank Allah for it.

[47] Compiler of this work Anayat bukhari, used to go to Masjid with his father in childhood.

[48] People who establish prayer regularly.

[49] This section is compiled after consulting the following material:

* Indian Journal of Psychiatry; The Islamic Prayer and Yoga, togetherness in mental health by Dr. Shabbir Ahmed Sayeed (Department of Medical Biology. Ibn e Sina National College for Medical studies, Jeddah, Saudi Arabia) and Anand Prakash(Department of clinical Psychology, Sina National College for Medical Studies, Jeddah, Saudi Arabia).

the entire body is very positive. It helps to maintain normal blood pressure which is a sign of good health.

Making intention for Salah, helps to improve this state of mind a step further. The act of intention itself is a declaration of Mussali that I'm going to retire from all my worldly affairs for a specific period of time. It intensifies the sense of protection in the Mussali from all sorts of worldly distractions and anxieties. During prayers he practically enjoys the relaxed state of mind which most of the mankind can only wish for.

Concentration of mind, through fixing eyes on a focal point on the floor, sharpens the vision. This physical posture has a direct connection with the state of mind which generates feelings of humility, modesty and piety. Psychologically, the Mussali is now in a virtual fortification, because all the signals coming from the brain are green, which are indicators on his piety and assures him of his innocence. This is such a strong clue to his impartiality that is enough to make him content by his feelings of security. He becomes more confident to realize that no one can hurt him as he didn't harm any one.

Recital of certain verses in salah; which includes Praise of Allah, supplications and refreshing commitment to faith along with Takbeerat is a practice which enhances the concentration of mind to a maximum level. During this act the Mussali becomes fully engaged mentally with such a phenomenon which provides him a chance to focus his thoughts on a single point – obedience to Allah. In fact this is the peak of mental relaxation in wakeful condition.

Allah Almighty has also enjoined the faithful in Quran:

> **O ye who believe! Seek help with patient Perseverance and Prayer: for God is with those who patiently persevere.**
>
> **Al-Baqarah 2, V 153**

Congregational prayers further improve this situation. Physical presence of community people on this occasion helps to remove all the psychological complexes, anxiety and stress from the minds of the participants and reinforce the sense of inclusiveness with complete security. Moreover, it develops brotherhood and fraternity in the congregation.

Ultimate beneficiary of all these psychological effects is the body of the Mussali. Relaxation of mind results in relaxing the body which makes the functions of different body parts and organs more regular and efficient. It leads the Mussali to physical health.

Musculoskeletal effects

Salah is such an act of worship which provides opportunity to the Mussali to move every single muscle and joint while performing different postures. It helps the Mussali to acquire maximum joint flexibility. Mostly stiff joints are the result of disuse and not of Arthritis. Despite such a deep rooted body movement it does not lead the Mussali to exertion. This is really a mild exercise but even then tension builds up in the muscles during physical maneuvers which get relieved by the spiritual ingredient – text we read during salah.

Musculoskeletal movements, when performing salah, help Cartilage to receive nutrients and oxygen. This unique living tissue otherwise, have no direct blood supply.

Exercise in the form of salah is at least five times a day with suitable intervals of a few hours. This schedule is excellent to obtain dual benefit. At one hand it provides mild but regular exercise and on the other hand intervals are suitable to relax the body.

Salah has psychological, musculoskeletal and cerebral effects on improving the muscular functions of Geriatric[50], Disabled[51] and Demented[52] patient in a rehabilitation program. The Physiotherapist

---

[50]   Geratric : adj. of or relating to the aged or to characteristics of the aging process.

　　　　n. an aged person who is disregarded as senile or unable to look after his/ her own best interests.

[51]   Disabled: referred to the people having either physical or mental impairments. It is a Synonym of Handicapped, which is now rarely used, and is considered offensive.

[52]   Demented: It is also known as Dementic dilemma. It's a loss of ability to decide because of the loss of ability to think. It's different from Alzheimer's disease, because it is not necessarily due to onset of age but more so because of prolonged idleness of the brain and repetitive non-brain mechanical activities in life over time.

of the rehabilitation center who assists the patient to restore and preserve joint range of motion through mobilization techniques and exercise may take this "prayer system" as a model for restoring the residual strength of the patient. Elderly people and disabled person can gain significant health benefits with a mild to moderate amount of physical activity, like the performance of salah, preferably daily[53].

"Evidence is also accumulating that those who perform voluntary prayer (nafal) can conserve and actually retard the loss of bone mass in the elderly, thus staving[54] off the ravages[55] of Osteoporosis[56] that afflicts both men and women. It is also possible to retard the aging process and confer some protection to health in later life. Those who have performed salah (Fard & Wajib), sunnah, nafal and Taraweeh prayers throughout their life get protection and a positive effect in terms of health and longevity. They reverse the life-shortening effects of cigarette smoking and excess body weight. Even people with high blood pressure (a primary heart disease risk) reduced their death rate by one half and their risk of dying from any of the major disease is reduced. They also counter genetic tendencies towards an early death. Hence salah (all) are necessary for Muslims to preserve life and their desirable qualities into old age.[57]"

---

[53]   Mohammed Faruque Reza, MBBS/ Yuji Urakami, MD/ Yukio Mano, MD, PhD: Department of Rehabilitation Medicine, Hokkaido University. School of Medicine Sapporo Japan

[54]   Staving: To break a hole in.

[55]   Ravage: to devastate; n. violent ruin.

[56]   Osteoporosis is a chronic progressive disease in which your bones become weaker causing changes in your posture and making one more susceptible to falls and bone fractures. Osteoporosis is a term derived from Latin that means "porous bones".

   Bones are at the strongest around the age of 30 but then they start to deteriorate. Essentially, if too much bone mass is lost in your later years or if insufficient bone mass has been accumulated during your formative years, you may be at risk of Osteoporosis.

   Ostelin.com.au; Osteoporosis and bone health

[57]   Physical Activity Guidelines Advisory Committee Report. By U.S department of Health and human services

   www.health.gov/paguidlines/report/default.aspx

Rakaat

This is a very interesting fact that the number of rakaat (units) in each salah directly coincides with the popular schedule of meals. Fajar[58] have four units as the stomach is empty. Zuhar[59] has ten units after lunch. Asar[60] four units as the lunch have been digested. Maghrib[61] has five units after evening breakfast. Esha[62] has nine units after dinner. Taraweeh prayer has an enhanced number of units as it is after breaking fast and heavy dinner.

This schedule of rakaat clearly indicates towards some wisdom behind it, to keep the body healthy in different circumstances of the day. According to a study:

"In Ramadan, after Iftar (breaking Fast) the blood Glucose level continues to rise from the food ingested. Just before the Iftar meals, the blood glucose and insulin level is at its lowest. After an hour or so after Iftar, the blood glucose begins to rise and also plasma insulin. Liver and the muscles take up the circulating glucose. The blood sugar reaches high levels in an hour or two and the benefits of Taraweeh[63] come into effect. The circulating glucose is metabolized into Carbon Dioxide and water during the Taraweeh prayers.

Thus the Taraweeh prayers help in burning the extra calories. It improves flexibility, co-ordination, reduce stress related autonomic responses in healthy persons and relieve anxiety and depression.[64]

Healing and Preventing Effects

According to some Medical experts, five daily prayers produce the same physiological changes without any undesirable side effects as those produced by jogging or walking at about 3 miles per hour.

---

[58] Fajar is before Sunrise.

[59] Zuhar is afternoon.

[60] Asar is late afternoon.

[61] Just after sunset.

[62] At night, before sleep.

[63] Taraweeh is the special prayer offered in Ramadan after Esha (night) salah. It consists of twenty rakaat (units) but some offer eight.

[64] Islamicity.com; The Medical benefits of Taraveeh by Dr. Ibrahim B. Syed (PhD)

The energy needed for the muscles during exercise is met by a process known as **glycogenolysis.** The rate of muscle metabolism is increased during the performance of salah. It results in a relative deficiency of Oxygen and nutrients in muscles. This deficiency causes **Vasodilation** – an increase in the caliber of blood vessels. It allows blood to flow easily back to the heart. The temporarily increased load on the heart acts to strengthen the heart muscle and to improve the circulation within the heart muscle[65].

Regular exercise in the form of regular prayers reduces cholesterol in the body. Cholesterol is one of the main causes of heart failures, strokes, Diabetes and many other ailments.

Regular salah is helpful in preventing indigestion through a course of light exercise.

Intention for salah directs the concentration of the Mussali on a focal point- the Creator, which is further enhanced by facing towards Qibla. It results to enhance the attribute of concentration on any desired issue. Certainly, with more concentration on a task, more aspects of the issue are revealed and broader vision is developed. Thus better results are achieved.

During Takbir Tahreema[66] there is an increased blood flow to Torso; hand and shoulder muscles which enhances efficiency of these parts.

---

[65]   Islamicity.com; The Medical benefits of Taraveeh by Dr. Ibrahim B. Syed (PhD)

[66]   Several Ahadis are there which describe the raising of hands along with saying Takbir. There is difference of opinion on its application but at the beginning of salah raising hands up to the shoulders or ear lobes is followed by all.

   A Hadis has been transmitted by Al-Zuhri as narrated by Ibn Juraij (R.A) (who) said: When the Messenger of Allah (Peace be upon Him) stood up for prayer, he raised hands opposite the shoulders and then recited Takbir.

   Sahih Muslim; Kitab Al-salat, chapter CLVII - 760

In Qiam[67] (standing position), the ability of vision is sharpened due to constant focus upon the point of Sajdah on floor[68].

When sitting in Tashuhad[69], hip, elbow, knee joints, back bone, wrist joints move to relax the entire body[70].

---

[67]   Wail b. Hujr reported: He saw the Apostle of Allah (Peace be upon Him) raising his hands at the time of beginning the prayer and reciting Takbir, and according to Hammam (the narrator), the hands were lifted opposite to ears. He (the Holy Prophet) then wrapped his hands in his cloth and placed his right hand over his left hand. And when he was about to bow down, he brought out his hands from the cloth, and then lifted them, and then recited Takbir and bowed down, and when (he came back to the erect position) he recited: "Allah listened to him who praised Him". And when prostrated, he prostrated between the two palms.
       Sahih Muslim; Kitab Al-salat, Chapter CLXIII - 792

[68]   It's forbidden to lift one's eyes towards the sky in prayer.
       Abu Huraira (R.A) reported: People should avoid lifting their eyes towards the sky while supplicating in prayer, otherwise their eyes would be snatched away.
       Sahih Muslim; Kitab Al-salat, chapter CLXXIII – 863
       In another Hadis the word supplicating is omitted. Anyhow, transfixing one's eyes in the sky is something which does not seem appropriate to the dignity which a man must observe in prayer. That's why it is commendable to fix eyes on the spot of Sajdah to keep it from roaming around and disturbing the concentration.

[69]   Abdullah (b.Masud) R.A said: While observing prayer behind the Messenger of Allah (Peace be upon Him) we used to recite: Peace be upon Allah, peace be upon so and so. One day the Messenger of Allah (Peace be upon Him) said to us: Verily Allah is Himself peace. When anyone of you sits during the prayer, he should say: All services rendered by words, by acts of worship, and all good things are due to Allah. Peace be upon you, O Prophet, and Allah's mercy and blessings. Peace be upon us and upon Allah's upright servants, for when he says this it reaches every upright servant in heaven and earth (and say further): I testify that there is no god but Allah and I testify that Muhammad is His servant and Messenger. Then he may choose any supplication which pleases him and offer it.
       Sahih Muslim; Kitab Al-salat, chapter CLXIV - 793

[70]   Abdullah b. Zubair narrated on the authority of his father: When the Messenger of Allah (Peace be upon Him) sat in prayer, he placed the left foot between his thigh and shank and stretched the right foot and

Joints host bacteria and viruses due to the fact that no blood cells and antibodies can get at them[71]. In an exercise[72] where joints are actively involved, blood flow gets increased which minimize the chances of joint problems – arthritis, painful joints and paralysis.

During Sajdah[73] (bowing down)[74] the brain receives a fresh supply of blood to get nourished and become healthier. It has

---

placed his left hand on his left knee and placed his right hand on his right thigh, and raised his finger.

Sahih Muslim; Kitab Al-salat, chapter CCXV – 1201

The sitting posture which has been explained above is known as Tawarruk. There is, however, one difference here and that is stretching of the right foot. The actual position is that the right foot is to be kept in a standing position, as in the sajdah, the tips of the toes touching the ground, while the left foot is stretched with its back in contact with ground and the open hand placed on the knees. Here the stretching of the right foot has been mentioned simply to show that if a man by any difficulty cannot assume this position with ease, he may adopt even this sitting posture.

[71] http://www.orthop.washington.edu/?q=patient-care/articles/arthritis/infectious-arthritis.html

University of Washington Medicine, Orthopaedics and sports medicine / Infectious Arthritis

[72] Salah is a perfect exercise for the joints and muscles. Almost every joint and muscle experience movement at different postures in salah. The repetition of these actions renders them to a kind of exercise of a mild nature.

[73] Sajdah- It's the prostration or bowing down on seven bones as is described in this Hadis.

Abbas (R.A) reported that the Messenger of Allah (Peace be upon Him) said: I have been commanded to prostrate myself on seven bones: "forehead," and then pointed with his hand towards his nose, hands, feet and the extremities of the feet; and we were forbidden to fold back clothing and hair.

Sahih Muslim; Kitab Al-salat, chapter CLXXXIX - 994

Abdullah b. Malik Ibn Bujainah reported: When the Prophet (Peace be upon Him) prostrated, he spread out his arms so that the whiteness of his armpits was visible.

Sahih Muslim; Kitab Al-salat, chapter CXC - 1000

[74] Abu Huraira (R.A) reported that the Messenger of Allah (Peace be upon Him) said: "The nearest a servant comes to his Lord is when he is prostrating himself, so make supplication (in this state)."

positive effect on memory, eye sight, hearing, concentration and the psyche. This posture helps to tone stomach muscles along with abdomen and kidneys. Spinal nerves are also nourished and spine becomes supple and flexible. Sajdah also prompts drainage of par nasal sinuses which decreases the chances of getting Sinusitis[75].

In the posture of Sajdah, knees form a right angle which allows stomach muscles to develop and hinders the flabbiness in mid section[76].

Sajdah enables fetus to maintain proper position in the womb of its mother. Many pregnant women are advised by their doctors to exercise this posture few days before delivery[77].

Human beings are propounded by electrostatic charges from the atmosphere which exudes perspiration in the Central Nervous System, which gets super saturated. Extra electrostatic charges have to be dissipated and discharged because it creates headache, neck ache, muscles spasms and some others. This phenomenon

---

Sahih Bukhari

It is also interesting to note that SAJDAH is something unique which is introduced by Islam in the prayers, as an act of worship.

[75] http://www.islamweb.net/emainpage/articles/159355/medical-benefits-of-prostration

[76] http://islamgreatreligion.wordpress.com/2012/05/20/science-behind-sajdah-prostration/

Science behind sajdah; by Dr. Muhammad Karim Beebani

[77] http://www.babycentre.co.uk/a544493/getting-your-baby-into-position-for-birth

Getting your baby into position for birth

takes place during sajdah[78] when the frontal lobe of the brain is lowered to the ground[79].

Yoga practitioners also believe in many of these benefits. That's why standing on head is also there as an important act in Yoga[80].

Turning head to right and left for salutation as to end the salah is beneficial for the neck muscles[81]. According to yoga it activates throat chakra[82].

Salah as a whole delivers an improved body structure[83].

---

[78] Sajdah has an immense importance in Islam. There are several Ahadis pertaining to its excellence. One is being related here:

Ma'dan bin Talha reported: I met Thauban, the freed slave of Allah's Messenger (Peace be upon Him), and asked him to tell me about an act for which, if I do it, Allah will admit me to Paradise, or I asked about the act which was loved most by Allah. He gave no reply. I again asked and he gave no reply. I asked him for the third time, and he said: I asked Allah's Messenger (Peace be upon Him) about that and he said: Make frequent prostrations before Allah, for you will not make one prostration without raising you a degree because of it, and removing a sin from you, because of it. Ma'dan said that then he met Abu al-Darda' and when he asked him, he received a reply similar to that given by Thauban (R.A).

Sahih Muslim; Kitab al-salah, chapter CLXXXVIII - 989

[79] http://www.ask.or.tz/viewtopic.php?f=69&t=2858

Why Sajdah in prayers must be done on earth?

[80] http://www.yogajournal.com/poses/481

Supported Headstand

[81] It's uncommon that a person who offers his prayers regularly will get the usual neck myalgias or cervical spondylosis as the neck muscles particularly become very strong due to at least 34 sajdahs, offered daily in five prayers.

Dr. Muhammad Karim Beebani

[82] http://www.yogajournal.com/search/?q=chakras

Yoga journal

[83] Although its effects surface with long term practice but its instant effects can be realized easily by a regular Mussali. He can feel the difference immediately after entering in the state of salah.

Salah and Yoga

In Yoga, activation of all the seven energy levels at least once a day is advocated to realize the true potential of the practice. Salah is less complex than yoga and is practiced ritually five times a day without any formal training is a boon to the Muslims. They get tuned to the energy chakras effortlessly integrating the practice with their daily routine[84].

Performing regular Salah[85]

It has also been observed that people who perform regular salah[86]; both mandatory and voluntary, retard the loss of bones mass in the elderly age. The loss of bones mass is a common phenomenon which afflicts both men and women.

The people who are perfect in performing all kinds of salah; mandatory, sunnah and voluntary along with Taraweeh prayer[87]

---

[84]   http://www.yogajournal.com/search/?q=chakras
        Youga journal
[85]   http://www.ummah.com/forum/archive/index.php/t-10462.html
        Medical benefits of Taraweeh Prayer, by Dr. Ibrahim B. Syed, Islamic Research Foundation, Inc. Louisville, Ky.
[86]   It is desirable to have constancy in doing acts of worship, including salah.
        Aisha (R.A) reported that the Messenger of Allah (Peace be upon Him) had a mat and he used it for making an apartment during the night and observed prayer in it, and the people began to pray with him, and he spread it (the mat) during the day time. The people crowded round him one night. He (the Holy Prophet) then said: O people! Perform such acts as you are capable of doing, for Allah doesn't grow weary but you will get tired. The acts most pleasing to Allah are those which are done continuously, even if they are small. And it was the habit of the members of Muhammad's (Peace be upon Him) household that whenever they did an act, they did it continuously.
        Sahih Muslim; Kitab Al-salat, chapter CCLXXII - 1710
[87]   Twenty or eight Rakat after Esha (night) prayer in Ramadan.

throughout their lives have better health condition[88]. A reverse impact has been noted in these people from life-shortening effects of smoking and excess body weight.

The more interesting finding is about the people having high blood pressure which is a basic factor of heart problems. Amazingly, death rate is reduced by 50% and the risk of their death by a major disease is also minimized.

These people also develop the ability to counter the genetic tendencies towards an early death.

---

[88] As compared to non-Mussalies. It can be observed by everyone, by visiting different Masajid. Most of them live a healthy life. Presence of a few sick people does not nullify the statement as mostly it is due to some other reason, if inquired.

SALAH; AS I[89] FOUND

Nearly half a century is not less to find most of the pros & cons about a matter, especially when it is not something technical and you are part of it; experiencing all the stages of this process. What was the level of my prayers, in terms of concentration and humility, during various years of my age, is the question which can't be answered by me[90]. But how much regular I remained in offering prayers five times a day, is the question which I can answer with my full confidence. I never missed a single prayer in my life, as I remember to the best of my knowledge. Definitely, I offered many of my prayers after the desired time but it was not left un-offered. It was only due to the blessing of my Allah who enabled me to do so with steadfastness. I don't have enough suitable words to thank Almighty Allah for this bounty on me. I also seek His forgiveness for this sin and beseech Him to allow me the competency to offer all my acts of worship, including prayers in a just and proper way regularly in future[91].

---

[89]   The compiler of this booklet, Anayat Bukhari.

[90]   Because it is a very private aspect of the matter which can only be judged by an absolute impartial personality – Allah.

[91]   Quran use the words of "Aqimu al salah", to relate salah (Al-Baqarah 2:43). It has wide meanings and the scholars are of the view that it includes regularity, punctuality and the observance of all necessary requirements for salah.

1. Organized Life:

Being regular Mussali means adopting a regular life style[92]. This is what I have been practicing throughout my life. I used to have scheduled my activities in between intervals of five daily prayers in a way which doesn't disturb the offering of my prayers with punctuality. It is helpful in maintaining a scheduled eating, sleeping, enjoyment and working habits, etc.

Schedule of eating prevents me from over eating which is indeed a major cause of many diseases. Eating three times a day allows me only the regular diet and keeps me away from un-necessary consuming of various drinks, snacks and other junk food. Mostly people become a victim of obesity by frequent consumption of these items.

Early to bed and early to rise is an ancient proverb and is best known for its positive effects. Full sleep at night allows me to take a fresh start every morning with a fresh mind and relaxed physical condition. It gives me the ability to perform my duties efficiently. Still it is a topic of research and many Scientists throughout the world are trying to explore more benefits of early rising. I have no doubt that I have been reaping its benefits since long. Some of them I'm aware of but many of them might be benefitting me without my knowledge. Al Hamd o lillah.

Many people have the misconception that salah prevents from discharging duties. According to my experience salah develops the ability to perform your duties accurately in an efficient way. For instance; I know that there is a gap of two hours between Zuhar and Asar prayer, so I try my best to finish my designated task in this time of two hours to reach for Asar prayer. Thus my working capacity gets increased by a fast pace. Moreover, I used to divide my time with the help of prayer times which enables me to do a variety of tasks in a day. Interestingly it helps me to increase or decrease the

---

[92]   It is because of the specific five times daily which change with the change of weather. In summer the gaps increase due to long days and in winter gaps decrease due to short days. As we are not supposed to leave a prayer un-offered so we have to schedule our daily activities in the gaps between five daily prayers.

time limits for a certain task in a natural way; as the day in summer is longer than in winter.

This scheduling works well to provide me enough free time to spend with my family, friends and certain activities for a healthy social life. I never feel any problem in discharging the desired tasks that are scheduled in my daily routine.

So, regular prayer is the best organizer of life. Regular Mussali never complains about shortage of time. Yes, this issue arises only when you are overburdened by the number of activities scheduled in daily routine.

Satisfaction of mind is the outcome of this organized life. I feel comfortable when I finish my day with all the scheduled tasks done properly. It is not less than a great bounty of Allah. I come across many people who are always in a hurry, running from pillar to post for the sake of one activity only – **BUSINESS**, still they can't. May Allah, bless them with contentment and relaxation by using this salah organizer. Aameen.

2. Flexibility:

Flexibility is one of the amazing bounties of Almighty Allah. We realize it only when one of our body muscles is pulled. The pain and discomfort we feel at that moment make us value the flexible body. To achieve and maintain this flexibility of the body most of the people spend a lot of money. Others who don't have money put their body to a variety of afflictions; jogging, exercise, etc.

The body of a child is most flexible as its bones are very soft and flesh is super soft but with growing age the same body parts grow stiff. In older age not only the body parts but also the joints become hard. Flexibility in the body is minimized and it becomes hard to move body easily in desired position. It is a common phenomenon but there are exceptions. Sometimes body remains flexible even in older age due to genetic immunity and sometimes it is the result of exercise.

In my case both of these factors- genetic immunity and regular exercise, are absent so I believe that I'm enjoying a flexible body due to salah. Regular salah along with other voluntary prayers has enabled my body to move freely more than many other people of this age. Alhamd o lillah! I consider it a great bounty of Allah who has bestowed this independence on my body.

Most of my fellow Mussalies are also enjoying the same freedom. Sometimes we see a few people in a mosque sitting on the chairs in a corner. When we investigate these cases, mostly we find diverse reasons behind their sufferings. Some of them are not regular Mussalies in young age. Some suffer due to workplace situations and yet some others are the victim of an accident. There is a very rare case when flexibility of the body is lost despite being a perfect performer of salah.

I believe it is due to the Barkah of frequent movements of the body parts and joints in salah which avoids stiffness of the joints and enables the body of the Mussali to move freely.

3. Weight control:

Gaining of weight is another serious issue with the growing age. Most of the people having tendency towards obesity put themselves on diet or tough exercise. In spite of this care many of them can't stop their body to become over weight.

I'm lucky enough to have a very balanced body weight, Alhamd o lillah. Although my eating habits are very organized and scheduled but being an ordinary man, sometimes I can't avoid over eating and lavish food. Despite it my body weight is in control. I believe this bounty is bestowed upon me due to establishing regular salah.

4. Shield:

Quran explicitly declares that salah restrains from sins:

> **Recite what is sent of the Book by inspiration to thee, and establish regular Prayer: for Prayer restrains from shameful and evil deeds. And remembrance of Allah is the greatest without doubt. And Allah knows the (deeds) that ye do.**
>
> **Al-Ankabut 29, V45**

I experienced these effects of salah in my life. Although in younger age my understanding of it was not so sound but gradually I started realizing that there is something that I'm unaware of, which stops me to indulge in sins. I started pondering upon it and came to the conclusion that it is a series of phenomena which leads to this stage of morality. I would like to share it for the benefit of my readers in a short form.

> ➢ Establish five time daily Prayer regularly.
> ➢ Regular salah leads to stay in the state of wudu, at least to avoid a frequent performing of wudu.
> ➢ To keep wudu intact, you'll avoid many things; too much eating, drinking, smoking, lying, backbiting, unlawful use of eyes and other body parts, etc.
> ➢ This habit upgrades in a certain time period in to avoiding certain acts like, use of abusive language, absurd talk, back biting, lustful acts and thinking, etc.
> ➢ After getting seasoned in this you'll further improve imperceptibly to a stage where you'll find yourself shielded against all kinds of sins in an amazing manner, in sha Allah.

No doubt, mankind is naturally inclined towards evil as is described in Quran:

> **Yet I do not absolve myself (of blame): the human soul certainly incites evil. Unless my Lord does bestow His Mercy: but surely my Lord is Oft-forgiving, most Merciful.**
>
> **Yusaf 12, V53**

Inclination towards evil does not change into reality by the Grace and Mercy of Allah when regular salah is established. My belief in this verse of Quran became stronger than before after observing it in myself.

Coming to the topic; how the body benefits through this practice, is now easy to comprehend. This schedule of habits keeps your body away from various intoxicants, smoking, over eating and drinks.

Thus, it helps to place a virtual shield around your body to keep it protected from unwanted things and actions.

5. Efficiency:

Establishing five times daily prayer helped me to practice an organized life by scheduling all my daily tasks and duties in the intervals between various prayers. This scheduling enhanced my efficiency many times. I used to do more number of tasks daily as compared to a non- Mussali. Even then I don't feel exertion and there is no stress on my body. My progress remains much better because I do these tasks with consistency on daily basis. It reminds me these verses of Quran:

> **Men, whom neither trade nor sale can divert from the remembrance of Allah, nor from regular prayer, nor from paying zakat, their fear is for the day when hearts will be turned about. That Allah may reward them according to the best of their deeds, and *add* even more for them out of His Grace: For Allah doth provide for those whom He will without measure.**
>
> **Al-Noor24, V37-38**

I believe that the word **ADD** in this verse alludes to the bounties like efficiency. Allah knows better.

UTMOST BENEFIT

How can we maximize our benefit from ablution and salah? It is the question which can be simply answered by saying; performing them with perfection. What is perfection in ablution and salah? It needs a little explanation.

a) Perfection in ablution:

- ➢ Making intention prepares the body to perform wudu in a way to extract maximum benefit.
- ➢ Using clean spot to perform ablution.
- ➢ Washing hands thoroughly by rubbing and applying soap.
- ➢ Applying Miswak for a few minutes.
- ➢ Washing cavity of the mouth at least three times and gargling (not when fasting).
- ➢ Blowing nose with putting water in nostrils up to the bone, thrice or more if needed.
- ➢ Washing face from ear to ear and from hair on forehead to the neck under chin.
- ➢ Washing arms including elbows.
- ➢ Wiping head, ears and back of the neck by using hands and fingers.
- ➢ Washing feet including ankles by rubbing them with your hand.
- ➢ The parts to be washed should be washed in a way that no spot remains dry.

➤ Pass small finger (pinky) of your hand between toes to ensure they are wet.

➤ Washing right parts first and keeping a sequence in performing wudu.

b) Perfection in salah:

➤ Making intention reminds the brain to get ready for entering in the state of salah by secluding from the environment, physically and mentally.

➤ Raising hands during Takbeer e Tehreema (First Allah u Akbar to begin salah).

➤ Keeping hands on the belly (men) or on chest (women) during qiam (standing position during qiraat).

➤ Keeping head level with the back during ruku (bowing down) in such a way that it makes a 90 degree angle with legs. Back should be straight enough to put a glass of water on it.

➤ Standing straight in qoma (standing after ruku) at its full capacity and contentment.

➤ Putting forehead along with nose on the floor during sujood (bending down) while both hands on the ground; pointing fingers towards qibla (direction of baitullah), putting feet on the ground by pointing toes towards qibla, keeping the parts of limbs separate so that they don't touch each other or belly (men). Women have to do sujood by observing modesty so they keep close their limbs to the body. Sujood devoid of putting nose and only forehead on ground makes a different posture which is not so beneficial for the body.

➤ Qeada (sitting position) is also different for men and women. Men have to lay their left foot to sit on and keep right foot erect in a way that toes are facing towards qibla. Both hands should be on their respective knees. Women have to do this in a modest way so they sit on ground by extending their feet on right.

➤ Focusing eyes down on the place of sujood during qiam and ruku while in the lap during qeada.

➤ Turning head right and left up to shoulders in salutation.

These are the right physical postures and actions in salah[93] and ablution[94] which helps the Mussali to follow the Sunnah (the way that Prophet Muhammad PBUH did) and to extract maximum spiritual as well as physical benefit from them.

O Allah! Grant us the wisdom to follow the right path and make our wudu and salah a complete spiritual and physical benefit for us. Aameen.

---

[93]   Sahih Muslim; Kitab al-salah
[94]   Sahih Muslim; Kitab al-taharah

BIBLIOGRAPHY

The following sources and literature has been consulted to compile this work.

The Holy Quran – English translation and commentary. Revised and edited by the Presidency of Islamic Researches, IFTA, Call and Guidance. King Fahad Complex for the printing of, Holy Quran

Sahih Al-bukhari – by Muhammad bin Ismail Al-bukhari, English online translation

Sahih Muslim – Imam Muslim, Translated by Abdul Hamid Siddiqi. Kitab Bhavan, New Delhi-110002

Jami Al-Tirmidhi – Imam Abu Isa Muhammad Ibn Isa al- Tirmidhi, Arabic

Sunniforum; The preventive and healing wonders of wudu/ online

Prayers; a sport for the body and soul by Mukhtar Salem

Medical benefits of Sajdah by Dr. Muhammad Karim Beebani

EveryMuslim.Net/ online

Wordpress.com/online

Turntoislam.com/online

The Medical benefits of Taraveeh; By Dr. Ibrahim B Syed

Physical Activity Guidelines Advisory Committee Report by US department of Health and Human Services/ online

Methodology manual for ACC/AHA guideline writing committees 2008

American College of Cardiology / American Heart Association

The Medical Benefits of Prayers (salah) by Arsalan Azad

Effects of Salat Prayer and Exercise on Cognitive Functioning of Hui Muslims Aged Sixty and over: By Bai, Rong; Ye, Ping; Zhu, Caifang; Zhao, Wei; Zhang, Jinfu

Social Behaviour and Personality: an international journal Vol; 40, No.10

Allah ki Itauat – Anayat Bukhari

Islamicity.com/online

The Islamic Prayer and Yoga; Togetherness in mental health – Indian Journal of Psychiatry: Dr. Shabbir Ahmed Sayeed and Anand Prakash

The Medical Benefits of Ablution - Ummah 1 TV/online

The secret of, Take a Bath for Health; Prasetio30.hubpage.com

Walnut Creek Chiropractor Blog| Dr. David Ritchie DC ; Sex and the Nervous System

www.myvmc.com/ lifestyles/female-orgasm

boloji.com; overmasturbation-cure Naturally, August 2014 by Dr. Vipul Sharma

UW (University of Washington) Medicine, Orthopaedics and sports medicine/ Infectious Arthritis

www.Islamonline.net; Ghusl after intercourse: why?